The 10 Keto Con
The Key to Impr
Fitness, Body an
the Ketogenic Diet

Table of Contents

What is Ketosis?

Ketosis is a normal - REPEAT - normal metabolic process. When the body does not have enough glucose (carbs and sugars) for energy, it burns stored fats instead. It's a process that your body goes through every day. Ever skipped a meal or two? Didn't eat many carbs during the day, or exercised for longer than an hour? Well by doing these things, you can initiate the process of ketosis.

Whenever your body needs energy and carbohydrates aren't there to meet the demand, your body starts increasing its ketone levels. When this happens, your body becomes incredibly efficient at burning fat for energy. It also turns fat into ketones in the liver, which then supplies energy to the brain. If carbs are restricted for a more significant amount of time (i.e. longer than 3 days), then your body will increase ketone levels even further, and with these deeper levels you will enter a state of ketosis.

However, most people are rarely in ketosis and never experience its benefits because the body prefers to use sugar as its primary fuel source – especially if you're constantly eating carbs and sugary foods and snacks.

To put it simply, the keto diet is a high fat, moderate protein, low carbohydrate diet that switches your metabolism to using fat instead of glucose as its primary energy source, which makes it extremely easy to lose weight and stay energized and focused while following the diet.

The 10 Keto Commandments: An Introduction

I've written these commandments as a guide to set anyone who wants to lose weight and increase their health, fitness, and well-being on the right path. They are also for the benefit of people who have serious health issues as the result of a high carb-based diet, such as obesity, diabetes, atherosclerosis, vascular diseases, and many more.

I feel that it is important to state that a ketogenic diet is a very efficient way to lose weight, but also it can and has changed a lot of people's lives in so many ways. So, whether your plan is to just lose a few pounds or to change your life, these 10 commandments apply to everyone.

So, here are the 10 Keto Commandments in order of importance; knowledge that every individual will need to initially reach the stage of ketosis and to start burning some serious fat.

Keto Commandment 1: Macros and Calories

Macros? What are macros? For those of you that are new to dieting or the keto diet, macro is short for macronutrient. Macronutrients are fats, carbohydrates, and proteins. Now, before setting your macros, if you are starting the keto diet to lose weight then you need to figure out your calorie intake goal.

For those of you who are starting keto for health benefits and other reasons, you don't necessarily need to set/track your calories, however you will need to set your macros as the keto diet is high fat, moderate protein and low carb, so without setting your macros you may never enter ketosis. Too much protein and you're doing the Atkins diet; too many carbs and you will just be on a typical low carb diet and will end up feeling very hungry and lethargic after a week or two.

So, first let's set your calorie intake. In order to figure this out, there is a simple equation using your height, weight and age.

First, figure out your RMR (resting metabolic rate). That's how many calories your body needs simply to function, not including any activity.

Using a calculator, work out the following using your weight in kilograms and height in centimetres:

Male: 10 x weight + 6.25 x height − 5 x age + 5
Female: 10 x weight + 6.25 x height − 5 x age − 161

Then multiply that number by your "activity factor":

- Newb: 1.2
- Beginner: 1.375
- Intermediate: 1.55

- Advanced: 1.725
- Active all day: 1.9

Finally, if your goal is to lose weight then subtract 20% from your figure and then you'll have your daily calorie goal. If you're not looking to lose weight specifically with keto, then you don't need to subtract 20%.

Here is an example of what the above should look like:

Andrew is a 33 year old male who weighs 90kg and is 181cm tall. He works out three times a week and has an active job, so would fall in the Intermediate category. So, to calculate his daily calories number he would type in:

10 x 90 + 6.25 x 181 - 5 x 33 + 5 = 1871

1871 x 1.55 = 2900

Andrew is looking to lose a bit of weight, so he would then subtract 20% from the current figure to get his daily calorie number, which is 2320.

I must add that if you are severely overweight or obese, this equation might not be for you. So in your case, I'd recommend starting your daily calories at 2500 for a male and 2000 for a female for the first month to make it easier for your body to switch into ketosis. If you are severely overweight, it's going to be a very big shock to the body to not only switch from a carb-based diet to a diet high in fat, but, in addition, the significant drop in calories would be a lot harder to cope with. So for you guys, drop your calories after the first month only if required, i.e. if you're seeing good results, there's no need to drop your calories at all.

Now you have your daily calories, the most important part is where those calories are going to come from, and that's where your macro ratio is needed:

- 75% of your calories are going to come from fat.
- 20% of your calories are going to come from protein.
- The last 5% are going to come from carbs (not just any carbs, but we'll cover that later on).

To track your calories/macros, the easiest way is to use an app. Given it's 2019 and you can't go anywhere without seeing them, I'm going to assume you have a smartphone. There are many calorie tracker apps available, however the most popular and easiest to use seems to be MyFitnessPal. You can use it on your tablet, phone or laptop, and there are a lot of tutorials online to get you started.

For those of you who really don't want to track any calories or macros, you can do the keto diet without tracking. All you need to do is make sure every meal you have is high fat, moderate protein, and low carb, and eat until you are satisfied.

Your body will tell you if you are going wrong. For instance, if you are hungry an hour after a meal, then you clearly didn't eat enough fat in your last meal; if you feel lethargic but have eaten enough, then possibly you may have consumed too many carbs, and as a result have been kicked out of ketosis.

I understand that just by reading the last few pages, you are probably feeling a bit overwhelmed with all the numbers and jargon, however you only have to figure out your calories once, then you can get on with the diet.

Keto Commandment 2: Fat Phobia

Now, most people starting the keto diet will have a fat phobia. They think that if they eat higher amounts of fat that they will get fat, but that couldn't be further from the truth. Fat doesn't make you fat and here's why. The number one hormone for storing fat in the body is INSULIN. When you have high levels of insulin, your body is in fat storage mode, and can you guess what spikes insulin? … CARBOHYDRATES.

Yes, carbs are responsible. Now, I am not saying carbs are bad, absolutely not, but to a person trying to enter ketosis carbs will stop you instantly. The idea is to keep insulin levels low at all times, and to do that you need to swap your carbs for fats. When you stop eating carbs, your body needs an alternative fuel source and that is going to be fats, so make sure you eat enough fat so it's easier for your body to make the switch.

It's been over 50 years since the "war on fat" began, so it makes total sense if you're still afraid to embrace it. We've all been taught our entire lives to avoid fat, but now you need to embrace it and enjoy those fatty foods as they are going to be your body's fuel from now on. Here is a list of foods you can enjoy:

- avocado
- sour cream
- heavy cream
- coconut oil
- olive oil
- real butter
- ghee
- full fat cheeses
- whole-plain Greek yoghurt
- nuts
- fatty cuts of meat, poultry, seafood

When you eat a delicious pork chop or steak, don't cut off the fat and just eat the meat, eat it all. You don't see crocs or lions in the wild killing their prey then leaving the fatty parts, do you? No, that's the part they want the most, because it provides the most amount of energy, and keeps them full and strong until their next kill or, in our case, our next meal.

You will no longer be looking for the low fat yoghurts, low fat cheeses or low fat spreads; you will be having the full fat ones, the ones that taste nicer, the ones that will provide you with the most energy and the most benefit.

One of the secrets to staying on track is to eat fat to satiety. Fat keeps us full and energized, so it becomes a sustainable way of eating.

To summarize:

- Fat doesn't make you fat.
- Fat is now your primary fuel source, so eat enough fat to fuel your body.
- Eat until you are satisfied.

Keto Commandment 3: Which Type of Fat?

Not all fats are created equal. Because fats are the whole foundation behind keto, you want to ensure you are eating the right ones. Which are the wrong fats? Processed fats.

Examples of fats you should absolutely avoid are vegetable fats and seed oils such as:

- sunflower oil
- soybean oil
- canola oil
- hydrogenated fats such as margarine

Most of the time, these are going to cause you a lot more health problems, like increased risk of heart disease, increased risk of cancer, and a spike in your LDL cholesterol (bad cholesterol) levels.

There are enough good fats in the world that you will have no problem reaching your daily fat macros.

To summarize:

- Don't fear saturated fats.
- Choose fats that are as unprocessed as possible.
- Avoid fats and oils found in processed, packaged food that was made in a factory.

After all, the purpose of the ketogenic diet is to improve your health and that includes not only maintaining the proper fat, protein and carb ratio, but also choosing foods that promote good health.

Don't go looking for microwave meals or quick fixes, as you will find they may have a lot of fat in them but that fat is processed and unhealthy. Cook or prep your own food, whole foods, and you can't go wrong.

Keto Commandment 4: Sodium/Salt

Salt is a critical component to the ketogenic diet; it is discussed quite frequently in the keto community and for good reason. Up until now, everything you have been eating on a standard diet has been salted out of existence. Did you eat takeaway food? Salted. Did you eat cereal? Salted. Did you live on energy drinks or sodas? Salted.

You've had so much salt up until now, you probably had no idea of just how much you were actually consuming.

After being told for so many years by the non-keto world that we need to reduce our salt intake, to be careful how much salt we use, and be scared out of our minds by advertising and doctors about the role of salt in the cause of heart disease, kidney failure, and other horrible-sounding illnesses, we need to readjust the way we think about and consume salt.

If we were still eating all the CARBage and fortified food, junk that is deliberately stuffed full of salt and a bunch of other minerals and vitamins, then consuming too much salt could become an issue. High carbohydrate consumption causes the body to retain water and salt. Even if you've been eating "clean", if you've been eating higher amounts of carbs (and that means any kind of carbs your body has held onto), any salt that has been ingested has stuck.

Now that you're living ketogenically, NONE of your food is salted, and because you are eating very few carbs and no fortified foods, your body is expelling electrolytes (sodium, potassium and magnesium) like mad. You must replace all the salt that companies have been adding to the food you'd previously eaten in order to avoid electrolyte deficiencies, which can be very dangerous. What all those doctors and experts forget to do while they're telling us to cut down on salt, is tell us that salt is vitally important for the body to function properly.

Like many things, if we have too much, it becomes unhelpful, but our body is very good at telling us if we've had too much if we're practised at listening to it. Also, in a ketogenic body, you're more likely to have too little salt than too much, and if you do manage to over-consume, it manifests in unpleasant side effects long before it becomes dangerous.

Salt (Sodium, Na) performs many important functions in the body:

- It helps keep our cells hydrated through assisting the elasticity of the cell wall.

- It assists in the uptake of potassium into our cells. If we don't have enough salt in our system, when we eat potassium rich foods, the potassium is wasted, because it doesn't transfer through the cell wall effectively.

- It assists in maintaining the delicate fluid balance in and surrounding all the cells in our body.

- It plays a crucial role in digestion along the entire digestive tract, from the acidic environment of the stomach, to the absorption of fluid in the bowel.

The body's response to too much salt is to address the balance in our cells. Our kidneys and bowel will expel the excess salt, along with fluid, which is where risk of dehydration comes in if people intake too much salt without enough water.

Because of the body's natural reaction to excess salt, it's almost impossible to ingest dangerous amounts of salt on a ketogenic diet. If we are fat-fuelling our bodies, then our body will not hold onto excess sodium. It is the process of carbohydrate-fuelling that makes excess sodium a significant long-term issue for the heart and kidneys in particular.

This is why, when we were pre-keto, adding salt to already salted, fortified, processed, ruined "food" was such an issue. Nobody told us that though, did they?

As "ketogenic lifestylers", we need approximately two teaspoons of salt per day. This can come in some of the foods we eat, like cheese and salted butter, etc., but it is also important to use salt as a seasoning.

Use unprocessed rock salt if you can afford it, such as Himalayan pink salt or Celtic grey salt, or iodised table salt if you're on a budget. Rock salt is the best option, but budget restrictions sometimes win out.

Did you know that every important Roman city was located near a source of salt, and that the average Roman consumed 25 grams of salt per day - equivalent to 10 grams (10,000 milligrams) of sodium? That's more than 2.5 times our current average intake.

Salt was considered so valuable that it was used to pay Roman soldiers and was a symbol of a binding agreement. In fact, the absence of salt on a Roman dinner table was interpreted as an unfriendly act, raising suspicion. It was the life-force of the ancient world.

If you don't add adequate amounts of salt to your diet, you won't poop, you'll have the shakes, you'll have heart palpitations, you'll get headaches, your brain won't function, and you won't uptake potassium, magnesium and other vitamins and minerals.

Salt is one of those minerals about which we have been fed one thing and told something else, without being given the information we really needed. Also, I feel its super important to mention that we lose a teaspoon of salt every hour we exercise, whether it be weight training of cardio. So, if you're not replenishing that salt, you will suffer on your keto journey.

In short: fall in love with salt, it could save your life.

Keto Commandment 5: Hydration

Water! Sounds obvious, doesn't it? But being hydrated and more importantly, staying hydrated, is key to enjoying the benefits of the ketogenic diet.

Even mild dehydration impairs memory, reasoning, and cognitive function, causes unnecessary fatigue, and makes you feel generally lousy. On keto specifically, some research also suggests that ketogenic diets increase the risk of kidney stones in people who aren't getting enough water. Not getting enough electrolytes can cause problems including muscle cramps/spasms, headaches, and constipation (this is especially true in cases of lack of magnesium).

Eating keto changes the way your body processes water and electrolytes. But luckily, once you know how it works, it's pretty simple to adjust your diet accordingly. Here are four things you need to know:

1. You need more water on keto.
Dehydration is a known side effect of ketogenic diets, for a couple of reasons. For example, on keto, you excrete more salt, as we know from Commandment 4. The more salt you lose, the less water you retain. At the beginning of the diet, many people also excrete a lot of excess ketone bodies, which is dehydrating. Basically, people eating keto need to drink more water to stay properly hydrated than people on other diets.

On the other hand, slavishly following specific numbers of ounces or liters can also cause over-hydration and electrolyte imbalances. The goal isn't to have as much water in your body as you can physically fit in your stomach; it's to have as much as you need.

A good rule of thumb is to drink until your urine is light yellow (although note that if you're taking B vitamins, this isn't a great guideline since high-dose B vitamins turn most people's urine bright yellow regardless of hydration).

2. Mineral water is a great "supplemental food" for keto hydration.

Mineral water is pretty pricey, so it's not an option for everyone. But if it's within your budget, even occasionally, it can be a great supplemental source of magnesium (a crucial electrolyte, especially for preventing cramps) and calcium (a mineral that's often lacking on keto, especially for people who don't do dairy).

For example, studies have shown that mineral water rich in magnesium improves cardiovascular health. Mineral water also has enough highly bioavailable calcium to reduce bone loss. Tap water and bottled water do also contain some minerals, although generally less then mineral water.

3. Starting keto or having cheat meals can cause massive water weight fluctuations – don't panic.

In your first few days on keto, you'll likely see a massive "whoosh" of water weight leaving your body. This is normal and it's not dangerous at all. Unfortunately, you do stop losing weight at that pace pretty fast, but it's nice while it lasts.

The explanation is simple: when your body stores carbs, the stored carbs also hang onto some water. In general, for every 1 gram of carbs you store, you'll store 3-4 grams of water to go with it. Depending on the size of your body and the amount of glucose that you're storing, this might add up to multiple pounds of water weight. When you stop eating carbs and burn through all the carbs you have stored, there's no reason at all to hold on to the extra water, so expect a lot of bathroom trips and a sudden drop in your scale weight!

On keto, even if you're being smart and careful to get enough salt, you'll also probably be eating less salt than you would on a typical diet. Salt causes water retention, so the sudden drop in dietary salt will make you lose even more water.

Of course, if you have one "cheat meal" and eat a bunch of pasta, you'll gain all that water weight back, but don't panic: you'll just lose it all again as soon as you go back to keto.

4. Tea, coffee, sparkling water, etc. are all hydrating.
In general, research shows that drinking things other than plain water is just as good – even caffeinated drinks are equally hydrating, in reasonable amounts.

Food can also provide a whole lot of water, especially really "juicy" vegetables like cucumbers (just think of how much smaller vegetables get when they're dehydrated). Some research has found that vegetables significantly contribute to hydration status.

If you hate the taste of plain water, then sparkling water, tea, coffee (within reason), or other beverages can also help you to reach full hydration. Just make sure you don't rain on your own keto parade by adding a bunch of sugar!

Keto Commandment 6: Veggies

Yes, vegetables. Can you honestly say you eat enough veggies? Well, now you've gone keto, that doesn't mean you can just live off bacon, cheese and eggs and you will be keto-adapted in no time. If you were to do that ,then you would suffer with numerous symptoms of keto flu (more about that later), which in turn will just make you feel like giving up and will prevent you from experiencing the amazing benefits of being in ketosis.

Like all of the commandments, this one is important because a lot of your nutrients and vitamins are going to come from veggies.

All foods are comprised of macronutrients – carbs, protein and fat. While meat and most dairy is primarily made up of protein or fat, vegetables primarily contain carbs. On a strict ketogenic diet, with fewer than 5% of calories from carbs, it's important to know which veggies are the lowest in carbs, particularly if your goal is to consume fewer than 30 grams of carbs per day.

On a keto diet, vegetables with less than 5% net carbs may be eaten relatively freely - have them with butter and other sauces! It is hard to over eat spinach, zucchini/courgette, lettuce, asparagus, and kale on a keto diet. These can be considered keto vegetables.

You will have to be a bit more careful with slightly higher carb vegetables like bell peppers (especially red and yellow ones), Brussels sprouts, and Beans, to keep below 20 grams of carbs a day on a keto diet. These types of carbs can add up. For example, just one medium-sized red pepper can contain 6-8 grams of carbs.

While tomatoes are technically a fruit, you can have them on a keto diet, but again be careful as their carbs are a bit higher and, combined with other foods, may take you up over 20 grams net carbs a day if you consume too much.

Here are two more general rules that can help you choose lower-carb and keto vegetables:

- In general, keto-friendly veggies are those with leaves. All types of lettuces, spinaches, etc. are good ketogenic options.
- Green vegetables tend to be lower in carbs than veggies with a lot of colour. For example, green cabbage is lower in carbs than purple cabbage. Green bell peppers are also somewhat lower in carbs than red or yellow peppers.

Vegetables and fat

Use keto vegetables as a vehicle for fat by seasoning cooked vegetables with butter or ghee. Better yet, sauté or roast them in lard, coconut oil, avocado oil, or ghee. If you eat dairy, you can make a cream sauce with heavy cream, cheese, and/or cream cheese. Another excellent way to add fat to vegetables is by dipping them in salad
dressings or other dipping sauces.

Keto Commandment 7: Exercise

Let me start by saying that you do not have to exercise to get into ketosis, so for all of you starting to panic, thinking "Oh no, I haven't got time to exercise, I'm too busy", or if you just hate the thought of exercise in general, don't worry. I've added exercise as a commandment because when you get into ketosis you will feel energized, focused and above all, healthier, and your mindset might change on wanting to incorporate exercise into your life. And when that occurs, you can come back to this book and back to this commandment and figure out what sort of training plan is best for you.

Regular, high intensity exercise helps to activate the glucose transport molecule called GLUT-4 receptor in the liver and muscle tissue. The GLUT-4 receptor acts to pull sugar out of the bloodstream and store it as liver and muscle glycogen. Regular exercise doubles the levels of this important protein in the muscles and liver.

This is a very important adaptation for maintaining ketosis because it will allow the individual to handle a little bit more carbohydrates in the diet, because the body wants to store them in the muscle and liver tissue.

Large compound exercises that use multiple muscle groups have the greatest impact on GLUT-4 receptor activity. This includes squats, deadlifts, push-ups, standing overhead presses, and pull-ups or pull-downs, or bent over rows.

Incorporating a regular exercise program that includes these resistance training exercises, along with running sprints and low-intensity exercise such as walking helps to balance blood sugar and improve the ability to get into and maintain ketosis.

Just be sure not to overdo it. Small amounts of high intensity training go a long way. If you over-train your body, you will secrete higher amounts of stress hormones that will drive up blood sugar and pull you out of ketosis.

Here is a sample exercise program to help:

Monday: Upper body resistance training for 15-20 mins.

Tuesday: Lower body resistance training for 15-20 mins

Wednesday: 30-minute walk around your local area.

Thursday: Upper body resistance training for 15-20 mins.

Friday: Lower body resistance training for 15-20 mins.

Sat/Sun: Recreational activities and walking.

I must add that if you don't have a set of weights or a gym membership, don't worry, you can do resistance training at home. Remember, you can use your body for resistance - push-ups and bodyweight squats are an excellent way to work out if you can't get to a gym, and there are some amazing at-home bodyweight routines online, so there are no excuses.

If you are a high level athlete or do regular intense exercise such as CrossFit, consult with your trainer or coach who is familiar with your goal to achieve a state of ketosis, and modify your training based on that.

If you are battling a chronic disease or have stage III adrenal fatigue, then I would recommend not doing any intense exercise and instead focus on stretching and breathing exercises such as yoga and tai chi, and low impact movement such as light walking or elliptical exercises.

Keto Commandment 8: Avoid Too Much Protein

Many people doing a ketogenic diet consume too much protein. If you consume excessive protein, then your body will turn the amino acids into glucose through a biochemical process called gluconeogenesis.

If you notice yourself coming out of ketosis, then see how you are responding to the amount of protein in your meals. Some people need higher protein levels, while others can do just fine on lower protein levels.

The key variables include your level of exercise intensity and type of exercise (resistance vs aerobic), and your desire to gain muscle or lose weight. Someone who does intense resistance training in order to gain muscle will need more protein than someone who is the same size and is doing aerobic or resistance training to lose weight. Another person who weighs the same but is only walking for exercise, will need even less than the other two.

You want to aim for about 1 gram per kg of body weight. So, a person weighing 160 lbs comes out to (160/2.2 lb/per kg) 73 grams of protein. When that person does heavy strength training (4 days a week), he will go up to 100-120 grams, but typically it is around 80 grams a day on off days.

Take your weight and divide it by 2.2 to figure out the grams of protein per kg of body weight. Aim to get this on your lighter workout days. If you are doing more strength training or trying to gain muscle, bump it up to 1.6 grams per kg.

Sedentary Individuals: 0.6-1.0 g/kg of body weight. If you are not exercising intensely, you may struggle to get into ketosis with 1 g/kg of protein, so try to drop it back to 0.6-0.8 and see how you do.

Active But Not High Intensity Training: 0.8-1.0 g/kg of body weight. If you are walking on a regular basis but not doing high intensity training (leaves you out of breath) or strength training, then try 0.8 g/kg and see what your ketone levels look like(more on that in the next commandment).

High Intensity Training: 1.0-1.6 g/kg. If you are training with weights or doing sprint-style exercise at least 3-4 times per week, then you will most likely need more than 1.0 g/kg. Try experimenting by bumping it up to 1.2 g/kg and inch towards 1.6 g/kg, and see how you feel and what your ketone readings look like.

It is ideal to get your protein in 2-3 different servings daily, with a minimum of 15 grams and a maximum of 50 grams per meal. The lower level is for a light weight individual while the upper limit is for a very large, strength training male.
Most of us should aim for 20-35 grams per meal. Here is an example of how this would work:

Individual A:150 lbs – needs 68 grams of protein daily. Does not exercise other than walking. This person should eat either two meals of 30-35 grams or three meals a day with roughly 20-25 grams of protein per meal.

Individual B: 150 lbs and enjoys doing resistance and aerobic training 3-4x a week but does not want to gain weight/muscle. This person should look to get 68 grams on non-training days and 75-80 grams on training days. So, 25-30 grams of protein per meal.

Individual C: 150lbs and does high intensity resistance training 4-5x per week and wants to gain muscle mass. They should consume around 80 grams of protein on off days and 100 grams of protein on training days. This would mean 30-40 grams of protein per meal.

Keto Commandment 9: Check You're in Ketosis

As we know, ketosis can be a powerful way to use your metabolism for weight loss, to increase mental output, and to improve physical performance. But how do you know if you're actually in ketosis? Fortunately, there are several ketone level testing methods available that you can use at home, like testing high ketones in urine.

There are three types of ketone bodies: acetone, acetoacetate, and beta-hydroxybutyrate (BHB). They each offer different benefits in ketosis and can be tested individually with ketone tests. Ketone bodies can be measured through your breath, urine or blood. You can buy most of these tests at your local pharmacy, making it convenient and easy to measure your ketone levels at home.

Track your ketone levels diligently while you're getting used to following a ketogenic diet. This way, you'll know how you react to different variables such as exercise, type and amount of food, and ketone supplements. Optimal ketone levels for specific goals can vary per person, so using ketone tests to know where you thrive is the fastest way to reach your goals.

Test High Ketones in Urine With Test Strips
With keto test strips, you can measure your ketone levels in just a few seconds.
When you have excessive carbohydrate levels in your bloodstream, your body secretes insulin and then converts it into fat. On a ketogenic diet, you minimize carbohydrate intake while increasing protein and fat intake, creating increased ketone levels and ketosis.

As you begin producing more ketone bodies, your body will need to get rid of the excess, which is excreted in your urine. Instead of being stored back as fat, the excess ketones spill over into your urine, and high ketones in urine are measured with the test strip.

Keep in mind, these test results aren't always accurate. The longer you are in a "keto-adapted" state, the more your body adjusts to high levels of ketones. Your body will optimize how it uses excess ketone bodies and they may not register accurately on a urine test strip, even if you are clearly in ketosis.

But, using urine strips during the beginning phases of a ketogenic diet can get you off to a great start. Key advantages of using a urine strip for testing high ketone levels in urine are:

Ease of use: Simply urinate on the test strip, tap off any excess urine, and wait 45-60 seconds for your test results.

Affordability: You can purchase a pack of keto ketone testing strips very cheaply.

Availability: You don't have to visit a lab or your doctor to see if you have high ketone levels. Find out if you are in ketosis in the comfort of your own home.

Test Ketone Levels With a Blood Meter
Blood ketone testing is the most accurate method for measuring your BHB ketone bodies, a critical ketone your body makes and ultimately converts to energy.

The testing method is similar to how people with diabetes test their blood glucose levels for high blood sugar. Prick your finger, squeeze a drop of blood out, tap it on a testing strip, and the blood meter detects your blood ketone levels.

Measuring ketone levels in your bloodstream provides the most reliable test results because it removes factors that can distort the results, such as how drinking water can dilute urine results. Your blood composition is highly regulated and shouldn't be affected by factors such as hydration, food consumption or becoming keto-adapted when you've been in ketosis for an extended period of time.

If the idea of sticking yourself with a needle gives you nausea, this might not be the best ketone test for you. Also, the blood test strips are a bit more expensive compared to the urine strips. This can add up depending on how often you test your ketone levels.

Assess Ketosis With Your Body's Symptoms

Listen to your body to estimate your level of ketosis. There are several signs and symptoms you should pay attention to. While not accurate enough to determine your specific ketone levels, they are a good gauge if you don't have access to a blood, urine, or breath ketone test.

Clear Mental State: Your brain constantly uses a significant amount of energy. When you are eating carbs, you may notice energy dips, causing swings in mental performance. When you are in ketosis, your brain rapidly uses ketones for fuel by utilizing your fat stores. If you are following the ketogenic diet properly, you'll be consuming plenty of healthy, high-fat foods, keeping your fat stores full.

Decreased Hunger: When your body becomes used to increased ketone levels, you begin using fat to break down ketones to use for energy. Because your body has a constant supply of energy, you won't crave food the way you do when your energy relies on carbohydrate stores.

Increased Energy: Approximately 90-120 minutes after you eat carbohydrates, your body has used up the available energy from the mitochondria in your cells. You start crashing, or losing energy quickly. When you are in ketosis, your body can perform well off your body fat, which is essentially a limitless source of fuel. This prevents a crash in your energy levels.

Increased Thirst and Dry Tissues: When you're adapting to a ketogenic diet, your body will be using up excess glycogen and you'll be urinating more. If you're not adding salt or electrolytes to your diet, you will probably experience some excess thirst and drier mucous membranes, due to lower hydration levels.

Avoid This Method

Some people have heard that if your breath is fruity-smelling, it's a good indication that you are in ketosis. This is not accurate; it may in fact be a sign of ketoacidosis, which is not to be confused with nutritional ketosis.

Ketoacidosis, or DKA, is a dangerous condition requiring immediate medical attention, and is seen most often in people with Type 1 and sometimes Type 2 diabetes. If you experience nausea, vomiting, are diabetic or at risk for diabetes, seek medical help right away.

Keto Commandment 10: Keto Supplements

Do you need supplements on keto or can you get all the nutrients you need from keto-friendly foods?

The short answer is that supplements can make your ketogenic diet significantly easier. It can be challenging to obtain all of your nutrition while also trying to focus on getting the right amount of macros, so that's where supplements come in.

What makes ketosis and the ketogenic diet healthy or not depends on the quality of macros and micronutrients (vitamins and minerals) you're consuming. To follow an optimal ketogenic diet, you need to understand supplements.

Why You Need Supplements on Keto

- The ketogenic diet is unique because it transforms your metabolism.
- Your default energy source is glucose from carbs.
- You take away this primary source of energy when you start a very low carb diet.
- Your body switches gears and shifts to an alternate energy source: fat.
- Your body starts ketogenesis: your gallbladder and liver release stored fats in your body, and, alongside fat intake, turn these fats into ketones, your body's alternate energy fuel.
- From being a carb-fuelled machine, you shift to being a fat-fuelled machine.
- This change is huge, and like all changes, it will take some adjustment while your body settles.
- Supplements help you get through this change with little to no pain.

- While not always necessary on a keto diet, supplements can help in three ways:

1. Reduce the Symptoms of Keto Flu

The keto flu is often caused by a lack of vitamins and minerals during the transition to ketosis.

For example, as your cells use up all the glycogen stores in your body, you lose water and with it important electrolytes (see Commandment 4).

Having the right supplements, such as electrolytes, can help prevent the nutrient deficiencies that cause the keto flu, and make your transition smoother.

2. Fill Any Nutritional Gaps in Your Ketogenic Diet

Because the ketogenic diet doesn't allow fruits and starchy veggies, you may not know where to get the vitamins and minerals you used to get from those foods.

Supplements make the transition to keto easier because they can give you important vitamins and minerals as you adjust to getting them from keto foods like red meat, eggs, and low carb vegetables.

For example, taking a greens supplements can be helpful if you don't like eating a lot of fresh kale and other leafy greens.

3. Support Your Health Goals

Supplements can support the health goals you're using the ketogenic diet for. For example, fish oil can support better cognitive function, which is a benefit of the ketogenic diet, while MCT oil can support your weight loss efforts.

Using supplements on keto helps you be at your best, and understanding how certain supplements work makes it easier to know if you need them. So, below are some of the most crucial supplements to know about on the keto diet:

Electrolytes: You constantly need to replenish your electrolytes, especially if you regularly exercise. If you don't salt your meals or eat a lot of leafy greens, then it will benefit you to invest in an electrolyte supplement.

Vitamin D: This is important for many bodily functions, including facilitating the absorption of calcium, a nutrient that could be lacking on a ketogenic diet, especially in those who are lactose intolerant.

MCT Oil: Short for medium chain triglycerides, MCT oils are a very popular supplement among keto dieters. They're metabolized differently than long chain triglycerides, the most common type of fat found in food. MCTs are broken down by your liver and quickly enter your bloodstream where they can be used as a fuel source for your brain and muscles. One of the richest natural sources of MCTs is coconut oil, with about 17% of its fatty acids being in the form of MCTs.

However, taking MCT oil as a supplement provides an even more concentrated dose, which has been shown to increase weight loss even further. A word of warning for first time keto dieters: use a small dose of MCT oil at the start as it can cause an upset stomach if you're not used to taking it.

Fish Oils: These contain omega-3 fatty acids which can reduce inflammation, lower heart disease risk factors, and help ensure a healthy balance of omega-3s to omega-6s. Omega-3 supplements can maximize the ketogenic diet's impact on overall health. One study showed that people following a ketogenic diet who supplemented with omega-3 fatty acids from fish oil experienced greater decreases in triglycerides, insulin, and inflammatory markers than those who did not. To boost your intake of omega-3 fatty acids through keto-friendly foods, eat more salmon, sardines and anchovies.

Exogenous Ketones: What are exogenous ketones? Many people starting a ketogenic diet have the same question. The short answer: exogenous ketones help you get into ketosis faster and support many of your health goals on keto. As we know by now, after you start eating a ketogenic diet and enter nutritional ketosis, your body runs on energy molecules called ketones.

Ketones are what replace glucose as the main source of fuel for your body. Exogenous ketones are those same molecules your body produces, except they're made as a supplement to help people reach a state of ketosis faster.

Exogenous ketones are supplemental ketones made to mimic the ketones produced by your own body when you follow a ketogenic diet. They can be found as ketone salts or ketone esters.
Ketones, or ketone bodies, are energy molecules produced by your liver when blood glucose is low as a result of fasting, carbohydrate restriction, or the ingestion of MCTs.

Ketones made in your body are also referred to as endogenous ketones (endo- means internal), while ketones made outside of your body are exogenous (exo- means external). It is important to note that simply consuming this supplement is not the same thing as following a keto diet, but it can provide great support to your keto diet, such as boosting your energy before a workout, improving brain performance, and increasing overall energy.

The type of ketone used in supplements is BHB, or beta-hydroxybutyrate. On nutritional ketosis, BHB is the main energy source your body runs on. When you take exogenous ketones, your blood ketone levels increase accordingly. By taking them, you can enter nutritional ketosis within an hour, especially if you pair them with MCTs (medium-chain triglycerides) from MCT oil or MCT oil powder. Exogenous ketones bound to salts, also known as a ketone base, can be dissolved in any liquid, so you can take it as any other supplemental beverage.

Keto Greens: Increasing vegetable intake is something that everyone should focus on. Vegetables contain a wide variety of vitamins, minerals, and powerful plant compounds that can fight inflammation, lower disease risk and help your body function at optimal levels.

Though not everyone following a keto diet is necessarily lacking in their vegetable intake, a keto diet eating plan does make it more difficult to consume enough plant foods. A quick and easy way to boost your vegetable intake is by adding a greens powder to your supplement regimen.

Most greens powders contain a mixture of powdered plants like spinach, spirulina, chlorella, kale, broccoli, wheat grass and more. Greens powders can be added to drinks, shakes and smoothies, making them a convenient way to increase your intake of healthy produce.

Those following a ketogenic diet can also focus on adding more whole-food, low-carb vegetables to their meals and snacks. While it shouldn't be used as a replacement for fresh produce, a well-balanced greens powder is an excellent and easy way for keto dieters to add a nutrient boost to their meal plan.

How to Start With The Keto Diet

So how do you start the ketogenic diet? You have all the commandments to follow, you just need to put it into practice. The easiest way to start is to do a little planning. If you have read this book and now think "Right, I'm going to start keto tomorrow", then you might hit a few problems, because it's a big change for the average person to eat according to a keto diet, and especially to immediately switch to a keto mindset.

What are you going to eat for breakfast? Toast, oats, cereal, maybe a croissant? You can no longer eat any of that on keto, so your biggest change on a daily basis will be your breakfast. Also consider your drinking habits. Do you take milk in your coffee? Sugar? That all has to change if you want to be a fat-burning machine, and if you want to be keto adapted.
I want you to run through a typical day for you - what you normally eat, what you normally snack on, and what you normally drink, as all of that will have to change. For example, you might usually wake up and have a glass of orange juice with some buttered toast for your breakfast. Well, not any more - you need to think about what you can now have instead. You might take sandwiches to work and some fruit for your lunch – again, not any more, you won't. anymore.

So, figure out what keto foods you like, find some good recipes and meal ideas online and you should be good to go. Keto is a commitment, and that is why I have written this book to help you. Everything you need to know is here. You can do it - and do it right and you will be amazed at the benefits keto can bring.

There is so much information out there now, as keto is becoming very popular you can find it all online - keto Facebook groups, Instagram profiles, etc. There are also some really helpful YouTube channels that show you just how easy it is to change your life and transform your body. One in particular is run by a gentleman called Logan Delgado. He changed his life with keto and has an amazing following on social media. To find him, search for "Goodybeats".

He has some pretty good keto snack ideas, too.

Unfortunately, this isn't a recipe book so that part you will have to figure out on your own. There are plenty of websites you can go to find amazing keto meals.

Here is a quick daily checklist to keep you on track. Write it down and keep it with you, specifically if this is your first time doing the keto diet.

1. Hit you macros: Remember, 75% fat, 20% protein, and 5% carbohydrate.

2. Salt your food: Salt is critical. Salt all of your meals, and remember that you lose a teaspoon of salt for every hour you exercise, so it must be replenished.

3. Stay Hydrated: Create a target and stick to it daily. I recommend two litres of water a day at a minimum, but the bigger you are the more water you need, and that goes for the more active you are as well.

4. Eat Your Veggies: Try and consume veggies with every meal as they contain the most nutrients - aim for four portions a day.

5. Exercise: Try to do some form of exercise or activity to get you moving. If you've been sat down all day, get up and go for a walk maybe.

6. Listen to your body: Your body will tell you if you're doing something wrong, i.e. you feel tired, thirsty, can't focus, go back to the commandments and see what you are missing. Perhaps you haven't been salting your food, leading you to feel very lethargic.

7. **Stay positive:** Remember, you can do it. You are in control and you have the power and determination, so stay focused.

About the Author

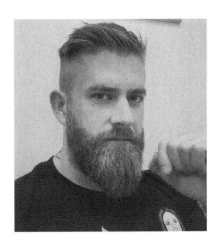

About Gary
Gary Corry is a family man with a passion for health and nutrition.
Since discovering the keto diet five years ago, it has been a growing
passion of his to help other people experience its benefits.

Thank you
A big thank you to my beautiful fiancée, Rachael and my children,
Logan and Megan
for supporting me in the research and writing of this book.

Printed in Great Britain
by Amazon